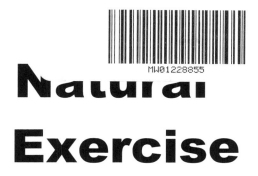

Natural Exercise

Basic Bodyweight Training and Calisthenics for Strength and Weight-Loss

Patrick Barrett

CONTENTS

Introduction   1

Breathing   5

Joints   7

Warming Up   11

Stretching   13

The Exercises   17

   Core   19

      Bridge   20

      Plank   25

   Lower Body Group One   27

      Squat   28

      Lunge   30

      Squat Jump   33

      Lunge Jump   35

   Lower Body Group Two   37

      Toe Touch   38

      One-Leg Toe Touch   40

      Sprinting   42

Pushing   45

   Pushups   46

   Plank Switch   48

   Dips   50

   Handstand   52

Pulling   55

   Pullups   56

   The Hang   58

   Inverted Pushup   60

   Climbing   62

What If I Can't Do Something?   63

Rest And Recovery   65

Reps, Sets, And Schedules   67

Basic Nutrition   77

Supplements   80

Vitamins   82

Working Out With A Partner   84

Conclusion   86

Books By Patrick Barrett   87

About The Author   88

"Walking is man's best medicine."

-Hippocrates, ca. 460 BC-ca. 370 BC
Ancient Greek physician, father of Western medicine

Books by Patrick Barrett:

Natural Exercise: Basic Bodyweight Training and Calisthenics for Strength and Weight-Loss

The Natural Diet: Simple Nutritional Advice For Optimal Health In The Modern World

Disclaimer:

INTRODUCTION

I would like to start by thanking you for purchasing this book. I know that your time and money are valuable, and I will do my best to exceed your expectations with the information you'll find here. We're going to cover a lot, but first I'll start by introducing myself.

My name is Patrick Barrett, and I have been interested in exercise and nutrition for as long as I can remember. I have participated in a variety of sports since I was a kid—I started playing T-ball and baseball in elementary school, then I played basketball and threw the shotput in middle school. My favorite sports were inline hockey (middle school through high school), wrestling (high school), and, more recently, rock climbing.

My first memories of exercise are probably from when my dad and my two older brothers and I would lift weights in our garage. I was in kindergarten at the time, which probably put me at around six years old (note: I don't really know anything about starting kids with weights at that age, so I'm not saying I recommend it or anything; this is just what happened).

My dad was a Division I football player, an outside linebacker/defensive end in the sixties, until a career-ending knee injury. He was (and still is) very strong—bench pressing over 400 pounds and squatting over 600 at 6'2' and 215 pounds. He knew a few things about lifting for strength, and so when my brothers and I started to get old enough, we would all work out together in the garage.

You might get the impression that my dad 'made me' work out, because some parents have that inclination when it comes to sports and exercise. On the contrary, I just knew my dad and older brothers were doing it, and that made me want to do it too. My dad gave me a basic routine to follow with pretty light weights, and I did it with them a few times a week.

I enjoyed the exercise, and I enjoyed the progress I saw. Off and on through elementary school and middle school, I would get up and do a light freeweight routine in the mornings before school, and soon I was playing high school sports and training through a combination of calisthenics, athletic conditioning, and heavier weight training.

In one of my first wrestling tournaments of my junior season, I wrestled an AAU national champion in the opening round. For those of you who are unfamiliar with wrestling, one of the main goals is to turn your opponent on his back, and one of the best ways to do that is to use his head and neck for leverage to turn his body. Well, this kid did a lot of that to me. He wasn't able to pin me, but since I was unfamiliar with a lot of his moves, I spent most of the match fighting off various attempts to torque, push, and pull my neck in various directions.

After the match, my neck was unbelievably stiff, which I did not think was too out of the ordinary. I wrestled several more matches in the next two days, took a couple of weeks off of wrestling for Christmas break, and then returned to the mat at another tournament in January. My neck remained unusually stiff, weak, and sore throughout this period (it was painful even to hold my head upright). By the end of that last tournament, it was clear to me that I was physically unable to wrestle at my best, and I went to a doctor. To make a long story somewhat shorter, I found out that I had a herniated disc and a bulging disc in my cervical spine, and that I could no longer wrestle.

Needless to say, I was not happy about that. Not only could I not wrestle, I was told that I couldn't do any exercise that involved lifting more than 25 pounds, and that if I exercised too strenuously or tried to lift too much, I could be temporarily paralyzed. Not something an athlete likes to hear.

Not being able to wrestle was bad enough, but feeling like I wasn't going to be able to keep myself physically strong through the type of exercise I had been doing since I was a kid was a very intimidating thought.

As a result of this experience, I was forced to adapt and improvise. I was determined to stay strong, and even to become stronger than I had already been. I learned about and experimented with a number of different bodyweight exercises, and after a while I began to see benefits from the bodyweight training that I had not been seeing with weights. I'm not going to say decisively and once-and-for-all that bodyweight training beats weight training in every area every time—that's a discussion for other people to have elsewhere. However, I will say that bodyweight training certainly has some advantages over weight training, and I began to see those advantages.

Over the years I've learned a few things about bodyweight training programs through experience, trial and error, and research on my own, and I've also come across some fundamental exercises that have shown me good, consistent results. My intention with this book is to show you those exercises, to teach you how to use them effectively, and also to throw in some tidbits I've picked up along the way which I think are helpful.

Obviously, we're going to look at some exercises—most of them you will have seen before, some you may not have. Anyone can write an encyclopedia listing every known exercise out there, but what's more useful is knowing which exercises provide the most benefit, and how to do them properly. These exercises work.

Before we get into those exercises though, we'll have a few short chapters covering some extremely important aspects of proper bodyweight exercises, and proper exercise of any kind: breathing and joint health (we'll talk about rest and recovery, reps, sets, and scheduling afterward). They are every bit as important to your success as the exercises themselves, so be sure to read them carefully.

I look forward to offering you the best advice I have on how to become—and stay—healthy and strong. Let's get started.

BREATHING

Breathing correctly during exercise is very important to getting the best performance out of your body, which leads to getting the best results from your workout. It is also an important component of optimal health in general.

In different time periods and in different parts of the world, deep, focused breathing has been connected to an incredible array of skills and benefits, from physical and sexual prowess, to better mental and emotional health, to long life, and even to supernatural powers like precognition and immortality. We'll leave most of those alone for the time being, but there is no doubt that proper breathing plays a huge role in optimal human performance.

As a general rule in exercise, you want to inhale on the easier part of a movement and exhale on the harder part. That means that on a pullup, you inhale as you lower yourself, and exhale as you pull up; you inhale when you lower yourself to the floor and you exhale when you push up on a pushup, you exhale when you stand up on a squat, and so on. Think of exhaling as a way to exert more power.

There are other situations, and certain more complicated exercises, that might require a more complex breathing pattern, but this will suffice for our purposes in this book.

It might feel unnatural on certain exercises, but you are definitely able to exert more strength on an exhale than you are on an inhale (and even more when you vocalize it —there's a reason for all that noise people make in sports and martial arts demonstrations), so even if it feels weird for you in some cases, work on making this breathing pattern second nature.

JOINTS

One of the biggest potential problems in starting any workout routine has to do with joint health. If you do almost any exercise incorrectly you can injure yourself—but the good news is that if you do them correctly, you will strengthen your joints along with your muscles and make injury less likely. This is an important thing to understood whether you're relatively new to strenuous exercise or not.

Many people run into joint trouble when they lift weights. Here's how that usually goes:

1. People want to lift weights to get strong.
2. A combination of ego and eagerness to see results leads them to use as much weight as possible.
3. They add so much weight that they aren't able to complete the exercise correctly, and instead of sticking with the right weight, they shorten the range of motion (ROM) and continue lifting.
4. If they ever think about implementing the correct ROM, they decide against it because it will mean not being

able to lift as much, and that will make them feel bad about themselves.

5. After months/years of lifting heavy weight through short ROMs, they attempt a real-life activity that requires full use of their joints (playing sports, moving furniture, etc.). Because their muscles and joints are developed incorrectly, they fail during this real-life movement, which results in injury.

Walk into any gym and probably well over half of the people there—even the ones who look like they're in pretty good shape—are doing exercises incorrectly, generally because they have shortened the ROM so they can do more weight, or more reps, and fool themselves into thinking that they're getting stronger. I recommend that you not be one of these people.

Bodyweight exercise is less prone to this sort of problem, but it's still just as important to learn it in this context to avoid injury, and hopefully to apply the same principles if you do decide to lift weights as well.

The first principle we need to understand is that we want to perform any exercise through its entire range of motion. It seems simple enough to understand, but few people actually do it. If you're doing any one movement in any given direction, you should continue that movement until you can't go any farther, in both directions.

Each exercise in this book will be accompanied by pictures at each end of that range so you can see what you should be doing.

What if the full range of motion hurts? Well, if you're lifting weights and it hurts, that means you're using too much weight, and you need to reduce the weight until it doesn't hurt any more, and then work your way back up over time.

If doing a bodyweight exercise through its full range of motion hurts, then you need to do a reduced range of motion, with the intention of increasing to a full ROM over time.

For example, let's say that you're doing bodyweight squats. Of course, a full ROM on the squat means that you go all the way down until you're actually squatting, with your butt pretty much right above your heels, and then you go all the way back up. Let's say that, even with no weights, squatting all the way down hurts your knees, and it starts around halfway through the motion.

In that situation, I would recommend squatting down until you feel just a bit of discomfort as you enter the range that starts to feel painful. On each rep of that set, come down to that same point in the ROM, and then go back up.

The next time you squat, try to work in just a little bit more distance on the way down—an inch, a quarter of an inch, whatever—so that you're going slightly lower than you did last time. In this way, as long as you're patient and don't push things too quickly, you should be able to work your way back up to the full ROM over the course of multiple workouts.

If you try this method and you find that the pain increases from rep to rep, or from workout to workout, you are pushing it too much. If you want progress, you must be patient.

This brings me to another critical point which is often overlooked by even enthusiastic exercisers. You can develop your joints in much the same way that you develop your muscles; that is, you can strengthen them, improve their performance, and lessen the chances of joint injury. The biggest difference is that it takes your joints more time to recover and strengthen than it takes your muscles, which is why you must also be sure to use proper form (which means a full ROM, among other things), eat right, get proper rest, and pay close attention to how your joints feel during exercise. This is absolutely critical for more advanced exercises like the one leg squat, or the one arm pullup.

You shouldn't feel pain in your joints when you exercise. If you do, make sure your form is right. If your form is right and you still feel pain, then do the exercise through reduced, pain-free ROM and work on increasing to a full ROM over time. Be patient. It pays off.

WARMING UP

It's very important that you warm up before you exercise for two main reasons—one, you will be able to perform better during the workout if your muscles are warm and your blood is circulating well, and two, you will be much less likely to injure yourself during the workout.

Warm-ups are not optional. You must include this step to stay healthy and get the most out of your body.

A basic warm-up consists of light exercise that involves and 'activates' all the major muscle groups in your body. Although there are many possible warmup routines that you can do, gym class classics like jumping jacks and toe touches are a great way to warm up.

Try doing a set of 10 toe touches (you'll see pictures and instructions later in the book) and 25 jumping jacks, and then repeat with a second set of each. The amount of warm-up you need will vary depending on your physical condition, how often you exercise, your lifestyle, what sort

11

of workout you're about to do, and other factors, but that should be enough for most people for these workouts. If you feel the need to add to the warm up, it can't hurt to increase the reps or sets of toe touches or jumping jacks, or even add some jogging, or running in place.

Your warm-up movements should be steady and smooth. Don't jerk your body or force any movement; the whole point of warming up is to avoid strains and that sort of thing, so you certainly don't want to strain anything in the warm-up itself.

As you get more comfortable with your regular workouts, you may be tempted to shorten or eliminate your warm-up. Don't. No matter how strong or fit you are, a good full-body warm-up will help you perform at your best and avoid hurting yourself.

STRETCHING

After your warm-up, it's important that you stretch (always do them in that order—you don't want to stretch 'cold' muscles, so always warm them up first). It's important for you to stretch out all the major muscle groups in your legs and your upper body. Your warm-up will provide a light stretch in these areas, and these more focused stretches will finish the job.

Here is a series of upper body stretches for your triceps, shoulders, and forearms:

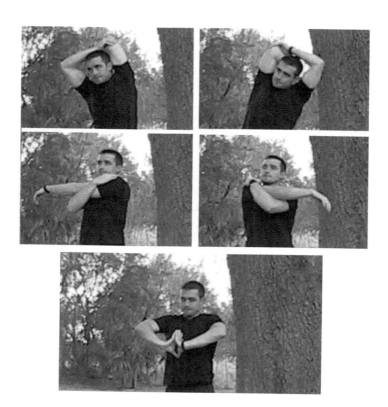

And a series of lower body stretches for your hamstrings, inner thighs, quadriceps, calves, and outer thighs:

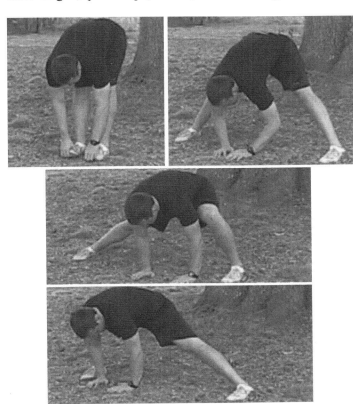

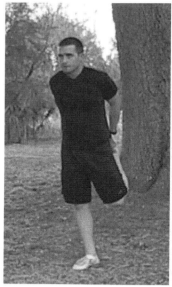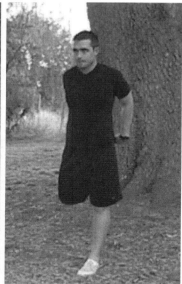

Assume each position comfortably, slowly, and smoothly. Sink as deep into each stretch as you can without discomfort. Once you can feel the stretch, hold the position for at least ten seconds.

There's nothing too mind-blowing or fancy about these stretches, but they have stood the test of time and they are an important component of a successful workout. They won't turn you into a contortionist or an Olympic gymnast, but they will keep your muscles supple and greatly reduce your risk of injury during and between workouts.

Just like with the warm-up, don't forget this important step. Every workout should be preceded by warming up and stretching, in that order.

THE EXERCISES

In the following pages we'll look at some of my favorite bodyweight exercises. Although most bodyweight exercises will hit most of your body, they also tend to focus more or less on one area. We'll be looking at them in four major groups: Core, Lower Body, Pushing, and Pulling.

We'll start with the name of each exercise and a short description, followed by pictures depicting each step of the exercise. Then you'll get any applicable notes and pointers, as well as instructions on any recommended variations on the exercise.

Some of these you will have seen before, and some not. I know that not all of these exercises will be new to you, but the point here is to learn and use a group of exercises that will give you great total-body results, and that means a mix of tried-and-true mainstream exercises, "forgotten" old-school exercises, and a couple of new and different ones thrown in.

Even if you've seen some of these before, think of this as a "rediscovery." Learn the form over again from scratch, and make sure that you always do it correctly. The results you get from doing an exercise the right way can beat the results you get from doing it wrong by 100% or better. Seriously. Very often, the difference between a person who sees results and a person who doesn't is just proper form, breathing, and recovery, even if they follow the exact same routine.

Spend some time making sure you do these exercises correctly, even if you think you already are.

One more thing—never start any exercise routine, this one included, without talking to your doctor first to make sure it's okay. Always listen to what your doctor says over what I say, and don't make any health-related lifestyle changes without talking to him first.

Now let's look at the exercises.

CORE EXERCISES:

BRIDGE
PLANK

BRIDGE

We'll start with this one, since it's probably the single best exercise you can do. Its builds strength and flexibility throughout your entire lower body, back, neck, and shoulders. I know it looks unorthodox, but it's an extremely beneficial exercise, and it's worth making the adjustment to learn how to do it. We'll look at it in two parts.

Bridge Part 1

In this variation, you'll use your hands to help out your head in supporting your upper body. Make sure you're doing this with your head on a thick carpet, a folded up shirt or towel, or on a mat of some kind. Let's take a look at the pictures:

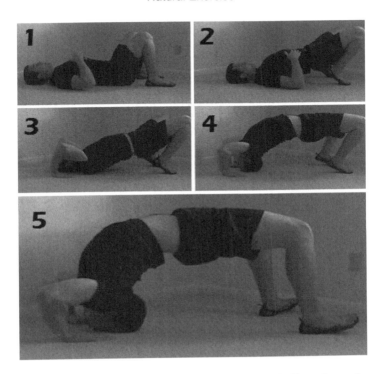

As you can see, positions 4 and 5 are very similar; the only difference is that in 4 I am holding the position on top of my head, and in 5 I'm stretching forward more so that my nose and forehead are pressed against the carpet. Your goal with this exercise is to get into this position (5) and hold it, stretching forward, for as long as you can. If all you can manage at first is the position in picture 4, that's good, just try to stretch toward something more like picture 5 with more of your face on the ground, as opposed to the top of your head.

You may notice in picture 5 that my toes are coming up off of the ground; this isn't a necessary part of the exercise but it may happen as you stretch forward onto your face.

Be sure to flex your butt and thrust your hips forward; imagine that you're trying to make yourself into an upside-down 'U.' In the beginning, you'll just want to hold the position and get comfortable in it. Once you start to get comfortable, try to support more and more weight on your head and less on your hands. Then, you're ready to try Part 2, which is really a correct wrestler's bridge.

Bridge Part 2

This is the same as Part 1, except that once you assume the position you will pick your hands up from the ground entirely, supporting all your weight on your head and your feet.

Just try the first version of the bridge (with support from your hands), take a deep breath, and as you slowly exhale, pull your hands up off of the ground so that your weight is on your head and feet. Be ready to put your hands back down if necessary; even holding the position without your hands for a few seconds is great if you're just getting started. Just make all motions smooth and controlled, whether you're lifting your hands, putting them down, or getting into or out of the bridge.

Try to hold the position as still and solidly as you can. Breathe deeply, thrust your hips up, and try to slowly increase the stretch in your neck, back, and hips so that you're rolling more and more from the top of your head toward the front of your face—you should feel pretty good about yourself if you can touch your nose to the floor and hold that position for 1-3 minutes. In the beginning, though, just holding the position on top of your head for five seconds is great, because it means you're getting

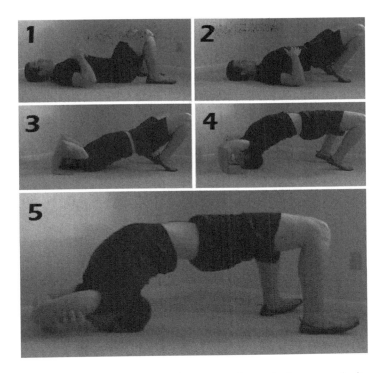

started. Work on adding a few seconds each time you do it, and stretching a little bit more, and the numbers will go up quickly.

I'm sure this looks strange and uncomfortable to most of you, but it can do wonders for your flexibility, your posture, and your neck and back. Speaking as someone who suffered a wrestling career-ending neck injury, this exercise can do more for pain in my neck in two minutes than an hour of massage, electrical muscle stimulation, lesser stretches, and pain meds can do combined.

You shouldn't try anything without talking to your doctor first, but if you're cleared to go, I recommend you get over the feeling that this is new and strange and just give it a shot.

PLANK

This is a great exercise that primarily hits your abdomen, and like many exercises, how well it works for you depends heavily on how well you do it.

Take a look at the pictures on the next page.

When you assume the position, experiment a little bit with relaxing and tightening your abs; feel how your midsection sags and lifts when you do it. Look for the optimal point in the movement where your abs are tightly flexed and you can feel them working and supporting your midsection; this is the position you want to hold.

Take deep, even breaths, and hold this position for as long as you comfortably can. If you want you can bend your arms and drop down to support your weight on your forearms instead of supporting your weight on your hands, just make sure that your body is in a straight line and your flexed midsection is supporting it. Doing it with straight arms will work your triceps, shoulders, and chest a little

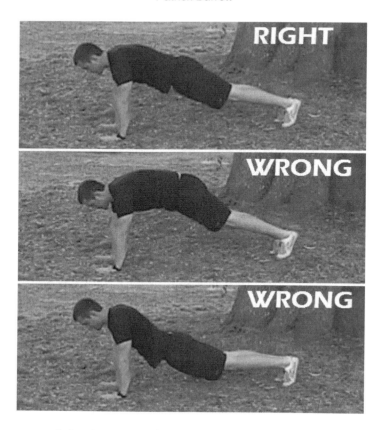

more, doing it on your forearms may allow you to hold the position longer and hit your abs a little more. Either one is good.

LOWER BODY GROUP ONE:

SQUAT
LUNGE
SQUAT JUMP
LUNGE JUMP

SQUAT

The squat is one of the most basic exercises there is. Remember to use a full range of motion.

Maintain good posture and a complete ROM on this exercise. High rep squats like these (100 or more) can be a great way to burn fat and build lean muscle, and bodyweight squats also serve as an indispensable warm up for jumping exercises. Stick your arms out at the bottom for balance, inhale as you go down, exhale as you come up.

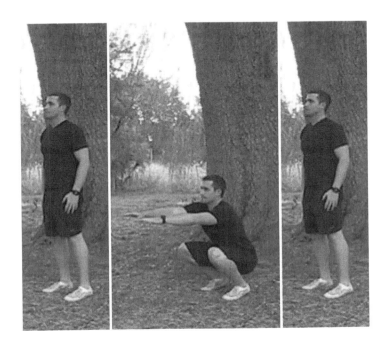

LUNGE

The lunge is a fantastic way to build your upper legs, and is probably one of the best exercises that targets your butt (along with the bridge).

Notice how at the bottom of the motion, your trailing upper leg is roughly vertical and your leading upper leg is roughly horizontal. Follow this form carefully, and lower your knee until just before it touches the ground to get the full ROM and full benefit of this exercise.

Of course, if your aim is to do sets of 10 lunges, for example, that means 10 on each leg alternating, for a total of 20 individual lunges in a set of 10 per leg. Always be sure to exercise your left and right side evenly.

Also, I recommend the "walking" lunge, where you don't just lunge forward and then bring your leading leg back to its starting position next to the trailing leg. You lunge forward, then you bring the trailing leg up so that you're a few feet ahead of where you were when you started. Then,

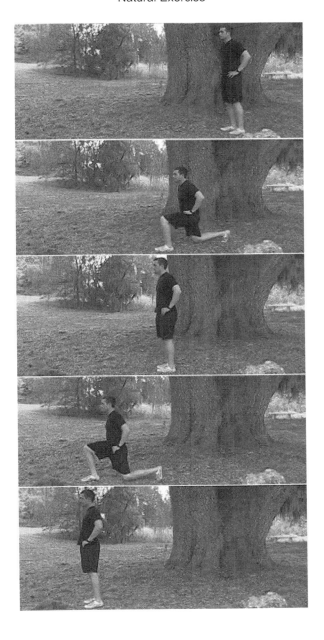

you lead with the other leg, bring the new trailing leg up behind it so you move another few feet forward, and so on.

If that's confusing, think of it this way: it's pretty much like walking by taking enormous steps.

It's best to do this along a hallway or in a field so you have plenty of room to move forward (although you can, of course, just travel back and forth along a shorter distance until you hit the right number of reps).

SQUAT JUMP

This is a pretty basic variation on a pretty basic exercise.

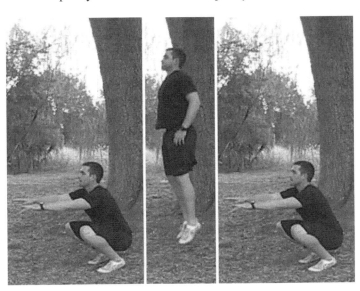

As you can see, squat all the way down as you did before, but explode when you come up so that you leave the ground. Land, squat down again, jump again, and repeat. I often use the squats as a warmup and the squat jump as a more prominent feature of my lower-body bodyweight workouts. This is not because bodyweight squats aren't great, it's because I am impatient and I get worn out quicker doing the jumps—if you enjoy higher-rep sets of the squats, by all means focus on those.

If joint pain is an issue at all, start with smaller jumps, or even leave out the jumps altogether and work on the squats for several workouts until your joints start feeling better, then try the jumps again.

LUNGE JUMP

As you might imagine, this exercise combines lunging and jumping.

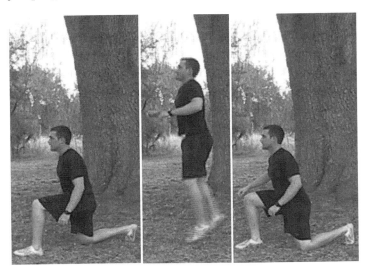

Make sure you get comfortable with this one, one slow rep at a time, before you try to do a lot in a row, because it requires a little bit of balance and coordination. Start in the lunged position, with one leg leading, the other trailing, and both legs bent so that the knee under your body is near the ground. Then press off into the air and switch the position of your legs, landing with them in the opposite position they started in. Be careful not to bang your knees on the ground.

As with the normal lunges, 2 jumps is really one rep, since that's what it takes to hit both legs evenly. Again, if joint pain is an issue, stick with the lunges for a while until this feels more comfortable.

LOWER BODY GROUP TWO:

TOE TOUCH
ONE-LEG TOE TOUCH
SPRINTING

TOE TOUCH

This is kind of an old-school exercise that's starting to make a little bit of a comeback—it's great for your hamstrings, butt, back and waistline, and it can fit in well in a warmup and/or a workout.

As always, keep your movements smooth and steady. Come into the down position deep enough that you feel a little bit of a stretch, but not so quickly or deeply that you strain something. In the top part of the movement, try to stretch your whole body and go up on your toes as you reach as high as you can.

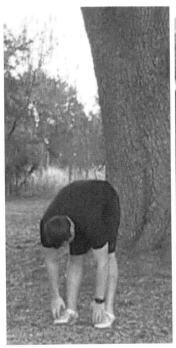 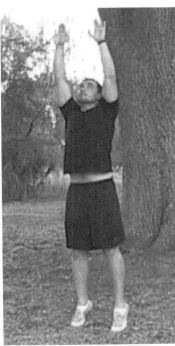

ONE-LEG TOE TOUCH

This variation makes the toe touch a little more intense and brings your balance and lower leg into play.

Take a look at the pictures on the next page.

Spend some time getting used to this movement, because it's easy to lose your balance in the beginning. Keep your legs straight and your movements smooth and steady.

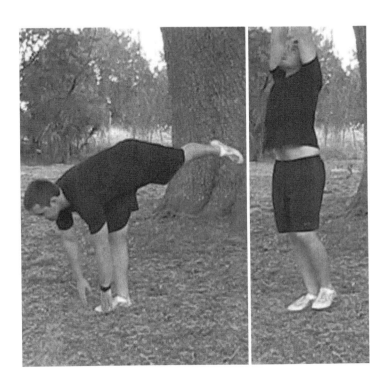

SPRINTING

Anyone can benefit from short sprints a few times a week, and I definitely recommend making this a part of your workout. Make sure you are thoroughly warmed up and stretched out (do your normal pre-workout routine, and also jog for a few minutes). If you're able to run in a field, yard, or park somewhere, pick a distance of around 40 to 100 yards, and sprint it as fast as you can.

Rest a couple of minutes, then sprint again. Continue until you can feel your speed start to drop off from fatigue. If it gets too easy, increase the distance and/or decrease your rest time in between.

You can also sprint on a treadmill if you need to, in which case you can just crank it up to a high speed (but nothing you can't handle) and pick a time (maybe 30 second to 2 minutes) to run—and definitely make sure you have at least a couple of minutes of a fast walk or slow jog before and after, for a warm-up and cooldown.

There are a lot of ways you can do this, but the two most important components are (1) do it at least twice a week and (2) when you are done, you should be sweating and panting. As long as those two things happen consistently you'll see progress.

PUSHING:

PUSHUPS
PLANK SWITCH
DIPS
HANDSTANDS

PUSHUPS

Used widely by military, police, and athletic organizations all over the world, this is still one of the best exercises around.

Many people are unaware of the abdominal development that pushups offer in addition to upper body development. To get the most out of it, do what you did with the plank—experiment with relaxing and tightening your abs, and find the optimal point in the movement where your abs are tightly flexed and supporting your midsection. As you do your pushups, you'll feel your abs working too, which will develop your abdomen and give you greater coordinated upper body results.

Exhale as you push up, inhale as you go down. The two basic variations on pushups are (1) move your hands 2-3 inches out from each other (this puts more emphasis on your chest muscles, as opposed to your triceps) and (2) move your hands in toward each other until your thumbs are touching each other and your index fingers are

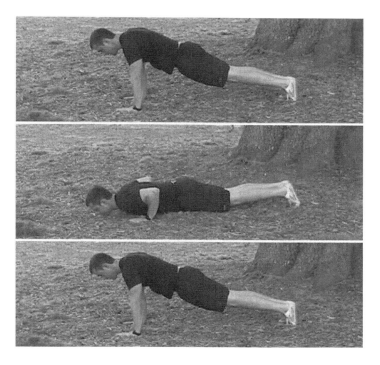

touching each other, making a sort of diamond shape directly beneath your sternum (this puts more emphasis on your triceps, as opposed to your chest).

If these are too difficult, you can do pushups from your knees—but if you do this variation, make sure that you're working toward the goal of doing the pushup correctly, and you don't just plateau and stick with the easier variation. The next exercise, the Plank Switch, will also help you get there.

PLANK SWITCH

This is a great core and upper body exercise for anybody, and especially if your pushup numbers are low and you still want a good chest and arm workout.

As in any exercises, proper form is key. Be sure to keep all the muscles in your midsection flexed as your rotate through the movements, and do so at a steady, even pace for best results (don't rush it).

Remember that two turns (one in each direction) is one rep, and always work out both sides evenly.

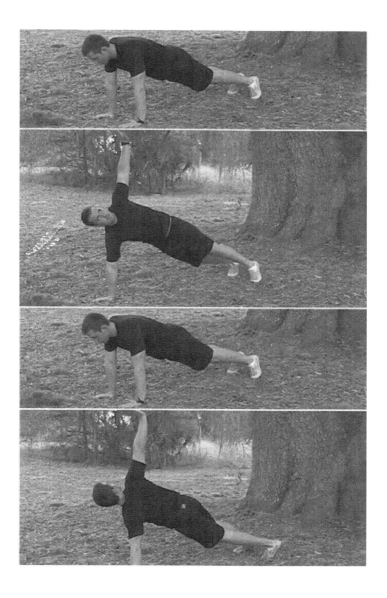

DIPS

These are more challenging than pushups, and they are phenomenal for building complete upper body strength.

Take a look at the pictures on the next page.

Notice the full range of motion all the way up and down. Getting proficient with dips will help you to develop a powerful upper body.

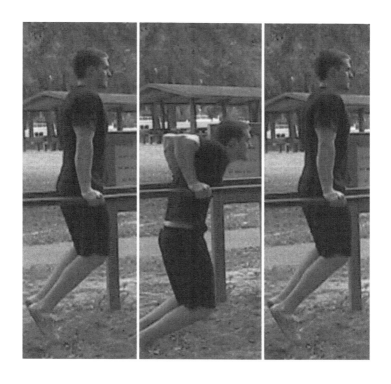

HANDSTAND

Handstands are one of my favorite exercises, and one of the best ways to build strong shoulders, arms, and hands.

NOTICE: If you are not prepared to tumble unexpectedly out of a handstand, do not bother trying to do one.

As you see in the pictures, you'll want to start on all fours, facing a wall, with your hands barely wider than shoulder-width apart and your fingertips about a foot away from the wall. Once you are in position, plant one foot on the ground and raise the other into the air, as pictured. Gently and smoothly press off of your bottom foot hard enough that you are able to bring the raised foot against the wall; then bring your trailing foot to rest against the wall as well.

If you've never done this before, it may be intimidating, but once you've done it a few times it will be second nature. Here are a few important pointers:

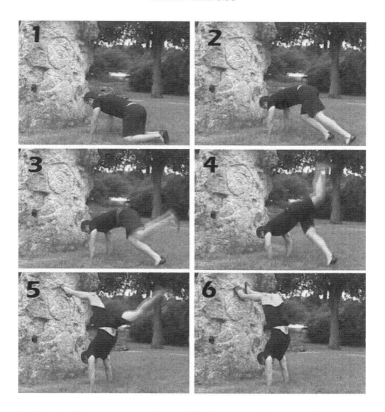

1. Don't focus so much on kicking up that you forget to support your weight once it's up there. Keep you arms strongly extended and be ready to support yourself.

2. Err on the side of kicking up too gently, rather than too forcefully. Just jump lightly off of the bottom foot and try to bring your leading foot up to the wall. If you can't quite get there, try again with a slightly stronger jump, and so on until you make it. That's much better than slamming yourself against the wall because you jumped as hard as you could right off the bat.

3. Don't try to swing both legs up simultaneously; you'll have much more control if you bring your leading leg up to the wall first and then follow closely with the next, as opposed to trying to fling both at one time.

4. Once you're up there, breathe deeply and slowly and stretch your whole body out; pretend you're standing on your tiptoes and trying to reach above your head as high as you can. Hold the position as long as you can maintain control.

That's it! A lot of these finer points will be very easy once you've done it successfully a half dozen times or so, but keep them all in mind in the beginning until they're automatic.

PULLING:

PULLUPS
THE HANG
INVERTED PUSHUP
CLIMBING

PULLUPS

This is definitely one of my favorite exercises. A lot of people avoid pullups (or perform them with poor form) because they are difficult... but isn't that exactly why you should be doing them?

The breathing on this might feel weird (in as you go down, out as you go up), but just concentrate on getting it right and you'll feel it helping you out. Be sure to pull yourself all the way up (if your chin hasn't cleared the bar, you are not all the way up) and let yourself go all the way back down on each movement for the best results. You won't be able to do as many reps as you would if you cheated, but doing fewer correct reps always beats doing more incorrect reps.

The top two pictures show a pullup. The middle two pictures show the chinup. The bottom two pictures show the proper grips for narrow-grip and wide-grip pullups.

As a rule, pullups target your back muscles more, and

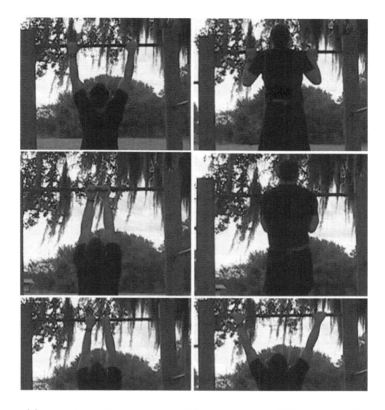

chinups target your arms/biceps more. When you do pullups, the farther out you place your hands, the more you target the outside of your lats, whereas the narrower your hands are the more your work the areas of your lats closer to your spine.

THE HANG

This is one of the simplest exercises possible, but it's still a good one.

Just take deep, slow breaths and hang from a bar or branch for as long as you can; this will increase the strength in your hands as well as your shoulders and back, and it's a good step to work up to the pullup if you can't do that yet (but still worth doing even if you can).

This can become an effective abdominal exercise as well if you concentrate on flexing your entire abdomen as you exhale—also, flexing your stomach will keep your mind off of your hands and arms.

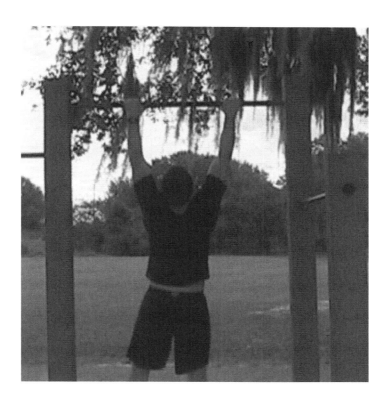

INVERTED PUSHUP

This is a cool exercise that takes a little bit of creativity to execute, but it's worth it.

Take a look at the pictures on the next page.

You can do this exercise in a gym, at a playground, in a tree, and at home, with a little bit of ingenuity. Ideally you'll have your feet raised to the level of your hands, but even if you can't make that happen, and you have to leave your feet on the ground, or just elevate them only a little bit, it's still worth doing. Concentrate on keeping you body straight from your feet to your shoulders, which is going to mean tension throughout your legs, butt, and lower and upper back.

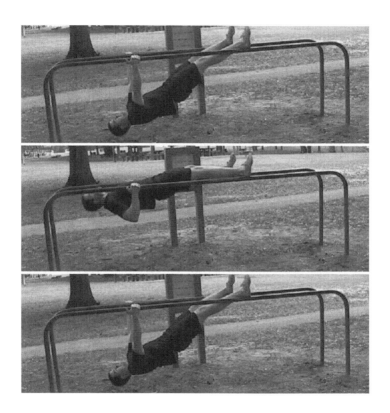

CLIMBING

Climbing is one of the ultimate natural exercises, although unfortunately exactly to what extent you can do it depends on your location. If you've got a local rock gym, consider getting a day pass, or even a membership. If you've got access to a climbable rope, climb that. If there are good trees or vines in your area for climbing, try them out.

WARNING: Climbing can be dangerous. Never climb to a height that could result in a dangerous fall without proper equipment, precautions, and training. Never climb up anything if you don't have a safe way back down. Always climb with a partner who can spot you, and could get help in case of an emergency.

WHAT IF I CAN'T DO SOMETHING?

Some of you will find that you are able to do all of these exercises. If that's the case, then great—keep reading, and figure out how to build these exercises into a complete routine using the information in the rest of this book.

If you can't do all of them, that's fine. You don't have to do every single exercise in this book to get great results, and you'll find out how to build a routine, which doesn't have to include everything, later in the book.

However, if you can't do something here, I would recommend that you make it a goal to do it. One way to work on an exercise you can't do is to hold a static position from the exercise for as long as you can. For example, if you can't do pushups, you can hold the up position for as long as possible, or the mid-range position. If you can't do a pullup, you can use a stool or a partner's help to get into the up position of a pullup—chin above the bar—and hold that for as long as you can.

You can also do negatives of the exercise. For a dip, that would mean getting into the up position and slowly lowering yourself into the down position. You can get the maximum benefit from this exercise by lowering yourself as slowly as possible, and by repeating it a few times each workout. For a pullup, that would mean again getting a partner's help, or using a stool, to get into the up position of a pullup, and then lowering yourself as slowly as you can. I find I get the most out of negatives when I take a deep breath right before and slowly, steadily exhale through the negative.

As you work on these variations, and continue with the other exercises, you'll find yourself able to do those exercises that were too difficult for you before. Above all else, don't be intimidated—through consistent hard work and steady improvement you'll be able to achieve your goal.

REST AND RECOVERY

It's easy to focus on the active side of exercise—which is, of course, the exercise itself. However, you won't reap much of the benefits of exercise if you aren't also aware of the other half of the equation—recovery.

Simply put, when you exercise your muscles, they break down a little bit, and your muscles feel sore. Afterward, your body rebuilds those muscles and they are a little bit stronger. You repeat the cycle over and over again, and over time you are able to become substantially stronger and fitter than you were.

If you don't eat right and get rest, though, your body can't rebuild properly. You will stay sore for days or longer, you won't get stronger, and you won't see any positive results. This is why it's very important to pay close attention to the way your body feels after each workout.

It's normal to feel sore for a longer period than usual if you're trying a new exercise, or if you haven't exercised a certain muscle group in a long time. Just pay attention, and don't jump back into that exercise until you're no longer sore.

After a relatively intense workout, you should expect to feel sore for a day or so, which is why the schedules (as you'll see) are set up to allow a day's rest in between more intense workouts involving the same muscle groups. This doesn't mean you can't ever get a good workout for the same muscles two days in a row, but if you do you should expect to be sore longer, and if you do it too often you will probably plateau.

You'll also see that some schedules are set up to have several days in a row of similar workouts; these are for more moderate workouts of shorter duration that will result in a lower level of soreness.

There are, of course, exceptions to this generalization. While everyone has to recover to improve, some people are able, through a combination of diet and training, to recover much more quickly, and there are elite athletes who train much more often than this. However, for the normal person, these are good principles to follow, and you'll see them in action when we talk about scheduling your workout.

REPS, SETS, AND SCHEDULES

Obviously, learning how to do each exercise is very important. However, it is just as important for you to understand how to set up your schedule for your workouts —that means which days you exercise, what types of exercises you do on that day, how many sets, how many repetitions in each set, and how long you rest between sets. It sounds like a lot, but it's not as bad as it seems, and like so many other things it becomes second nature once you do it for a little while.

If you exercise too often and don't allow yourself enough time to recover, you'll get run down and plateau, or even perform worse than you did before. If you exercise too infrequently, you won't see any results and you'll get bored, which will also ultimately lead to failure. You need to find the right combination that works best for you, which will really only take some basic understanding, a little trial and error, and a little paying attention—nothing too scary.

Now, I will provide you with sample schedules, but it's very important to understand that these are just guidelines. Many people have gotten to be in extremely good shape by following a wide variety of different schedules, and you don't have to follow these precisely. The best thing would be for you to get a sense of how to build a schedule on your own, but that will probably start with following an existing schedule and then modifying it once you feel comfortable with it.

Having said that, some people will just want a set schedule to follow anyway, so we'll get to that soon :)

Let's start with how many days per week you'll exercise. As a general rule I'd recommend 3-6 days per week of maybe 45-90 minutes of exercise. This is not a hard and fast rule—if you have good results following another schedule, then be my guest—but it's good advice for most people in most situations.

Also, as a general rule, you don't want to do strenuous workouts of the same type two days in a row—for example, if you do an intense pushing workout on Tuesday, you wouldn't do another one on Wednesday. Allowing your body to recover properly is key to your success, which as previously discussed means scheduling right and monitoring your own soreness.

Let's look at some specific schemes of reps and sets, and then we'll talk about how to use them in a schedule.

1 High Rep Set

Some people swear by doing simply one set of a high number of reps of a given exercise—for example, one set of 50 or 100 pushups five days a week. This can be effective if done consistently and with a high enough number of reps that it is challenging, and it also is very easy to fit into a busy schedule.

3-5 Mid Rep Sets

This is probably the most common type of scheme. In this situation, you will decide to do three, four, or five sets of a set number of reps. You might do three sets of 25 pushups, or four sets of 8 pullups, or five sets of 10 dips, for example. It takes a little more time than just doing one set, but it can also generally lead to a more intense workout since you go back to the same exercise multiple times. For this type of workout I'd recommend waiting around 90 seconds between sets.

8-10 Low Rep Sets

You will apply this type of scheme to exercises that you can't do too many of—let's say four or fewer reps. For example, if you can only do one pullup, or three pushups, you will want to try to get in more sets; that way you can get your numbers higher and ultimately do more at one time. For this type of workout, you may need to wait a few minutes between sets so that you'll be able to complete the exercise again—you might even just want to space it out through the day. For example, if you can only do two pullups, then do your two pullups at least ten times throughout the day, whenever you think of it. You'll start to be able to do more reps at a time more quickly than you think.

This takes more time for each workout, but you only really need to do it when you're getting used to a new exercise. Once you can do five or more of something, you can start doing 3-5 sets and increase your reps from there.

Ladders/Pyramids

These go by different names according to different people, but they are a great conditioning tool no matter what you call them. They're pretty simple: basically, you do one rep of an exercise. Then, you do two. Then, you do three—then four, then five, and so on, and you see how high you can go. Pretty straightforward.

People frequently do these with a partner. For example, you might do one pushup. Then, you get up, and your partner does one pushup. You get down and do two, then you get up and your partner does two, and so on. That way you get a brief rest while your partner works. If you don't have a partner to do this with, get a stop watch or just count off one second for each rep you just did (one second break after one pushup, then a two second break after two pushups, then a three second break after three pushups, and so on).

Usually, a ladder is when you keep going up until you fail, which might look like the following number of reps:

1,2,3,4,5,6,7,8,9,10,11,12,13,14,7

In that case, you would have done 14 sets successfully and then failed on the fifteenth by only hitting 7.

A pyramid is usually when you pick a number to go up to, and then you just go back down afterwards. That might look like this:

1,2,3,4,5,6,7,8,9,10,9,8,7,6,5,4,3,2,1

You could also do the ladder until you fail, and then do the pyramid back down. To use the first example, that would look like this:

1,2,3,4,5,6,7,8,9,10,11,12,13,14,7,6,5,4,3,2,1

In that situation, you did the ladder successfully until your fifteenth set, when you only hit seven. Then, from seven, you followed the pyramid back down, doing 6, 5, 4, 3, 2, and then 1.

Ladders and pyramids are a great way to mix up your routine, and also to get you to do more reps than you might have realized you could do. Two variations include counting by twos or another number (2,4,6,8 and so on instead of 1,2,3,4) and starting at a higher number than just one (5,6,7,8,9 and so on instead of 1,2,3,4,5). Those can help when starting at one, or going by one, gets a little too easy.

So, by now you should have a basic idea of how to structure your sets and reps. But how do you pick the number of reps to do in the set? Well, we're going to base that roughly off of how many total reps of an exercise you can do in one set.

If you can do less than five of something, then you're obviously going to follow the pattern of 8-10 low rep sets for that exercise, as described previously.

After that, it's not quite as clear-cut, but here are some general guidelines:

Once you can do five reps of a certain exercise, you should jump to five sets of your five reps with about 90 seconds in between, as described previously. When you can successfully get five sets of five reps with 90 seconds of rest in between the sets, try for five sets of 6 reps for your next workout, then five sets of 7, and so on.

Once you start to get somewhere in the 10+ reps per set range, you might drop a set or two and start doing three or four sets of a higher number of reps. At that point, you can decide if you want to focus on more sets of not as many reps (this will tend to make you stronger and increase muscle size), or fewer sets of more reps (this will tend to increase endurance and fat loss).

Any combination is going to increase strength and endurance, and build muscle and burn fat, it's just a question of tending more toward one or the other.

So that takes care of sets and reps. Now what about building that into a complete schedule? Like I said, there are many different schedules that you can follow and still see great results—as long as you are challenging and pushing yourself consistently, actually following the schedule will matter a lot more than what specific schedule you choose.

First of all we want to choose some exercises. There's some flexibility here; for best results I would recommend that you do most or all of the exercises, but if it's more realistic that you only do a few, then that's fine (you'll get better results sticking to a decent routine than you will giving up on an excellent one). You'll need to pick at least one exercise from each of these groups—you might pick one if you've never really done regular exercise, or haven't in a while. For best results pick at least two from each group, and the more ambitious among you can do more or all for the most intense workout.

Lower Body Group 1	Lower Body Group 2
Squat	Toe Touch
Lunge	One-Leg Toe Touch
Squat Jump	Sprinting
Lunge Jump	
Pushing	**Pulling**
Pushups	Pullups
Plank Switch	The Hang
Dips	Inverted Pushup
Handstands	Climbing

On top of those exercises, you'll be doing both the plank and the bridge, one set each for as long as you can comfortably and correctly hold the position, each day you work out.

We'll look at three basic schedules. Unless otherwise indicated, assume that for each exercise listed you'll do 3-5 mid-rep sets (or 8-10 low rep sets if you haven't made it to 3-5 mid rep yet).

Also, of course, assume you've done your warm-up and stretching before each workout.

Schedule 1: MWF

This is a three day a week workout where you do exercises from each group on each of the three days. It doesn't have to be Monday, Wednesday, Friday, but you do want a day of rest in between each workout.

Sun	Mon	Tue	Wed	Thu	Fri	Sat
Rest	L1, L2 Ps, Pl	Rest	L1, L2 Ps, Pl	Rest	L1, L2 Ps, Pl	Rest

Schedule 2 MTWRF

This is a five day a week schedule, where you do exercises from each group each of the five days, but you only do one high-rep set of each. You can arrange it so you have two consecutive days off, or two individual days off, however you like.

Sun	Mon	Tue	Wed	Thu	Fri	Sat
Rest	L1, L2 Ps, Pl	L1, L2 Ps, Pl	L1, L2 Ps, Pl	L1, L2 Ps, Pl	L1, L2 Ps, Pl	Rest

Schedule 3 MTWRFS

This is a six day a week schedule where you do exercises from one group of lower body exercises and one group of upper body exercises each day, and then you switch to the other lower body and other upper body exercise groups the next day.

Sun	Mon	Tue	Wed	Thu	Fri	Sat
Rest	L1, Pl	L2, Ps,	L1, Pl	L2, Ps,	L1, Pl	L2, Ps,

You may choose to start with one exercise from each group and then add exercises as the workout becomes too easy.

Like I said, these schedules are jumping-off points—once you go with one for a few weeks, you may add or subtract a day or an exercise here or there, or you may come up with your own schedule altogether. You can also decide to group all the lower body exercises together on one day, and all the upper body exercises together on an alternating day. As long as you are seeing good results and getting stronger without any joint issues, you're on the right track.

If you're relatively new to this kind of exercise, this might seem like a lot of information to keep straight, but it really comes down to the simple principle that you want to work hard and exercise, and then you want your body to recover so you can work hard and exercise some more. I'll leave you with two thoughts to bear in mind:

One comes from Bob Hoffman, founder of York Barbell and the father of modern weightlifting. He said that the most important characteristic of any workout is the "three Ps:" Puff, Pant, and Perspire. Any workout that causes you to puff, pant, and perspire will produce results, and one that doesn't, won't. Incidentally, this is why it's so important for you to be honest with yourself in following these schedules—once it gets too easy, make it harder. Add sets, add reps, and add exercises when things get too easy so you make sure you're always working harder and progressing.

The other thought is about two of the most versatile and physically impressive athletes of the modern era: Herschel Walker and Bo Jackson. Both men are renowned, even among elite athletes, for their physical prowess. Both men grew up knowing little about physical training, and just started doing a combination of pushups, situps, pullups, sprinting, and jumping. Their numbers increased as they exercised consistently, even fanatically, and each has left an unbelievable legacy in the athletic world.

The bottom line is they didn't 'know anything' about training when they started, they were just kids who worked their asses off and then ranked among the fittest in the world, ever. Some people like to mention their 'genetic advantages,' but I would simply point out that 'genetic advantages' seem to follow those people who happen to train consistently and intensely.

Pick a schedule, make sure you're working hard when you exercise, and make sure you recover when you're done. Then repeat.

BASIC NUTRITION

Nutrition is not complicated. Look at every animal in the world—they all know what to eat without thinking about it.

We don't know what to eat because we try too hard, and we think too much.

Good nutrition doesn't mean thinking about calories, carbs, grams of anything, or anything else along those lines. It's about eating quality, wholesome food. You should never go out of your way to stuff yourself, but don't ever feel bad about filling up on high quality fresh foods.

Make sure you see the 'bigger picture' with your diet—don't try to analyze every molecule that enters your body, or trick your body with precisely engineered cocktails.

Eat food in as close to its natural state as possible. That sounds kind of general, I know, so I'll get more specific.

1. Don't eat anything you could not have found somewhere 100 years ago. If you need a factory to make it, it's not natural, and it's not supposed to be in your body. This includes:

* 'nutrition bars'
* vegetable seed oils and 'spreads'
* highly processed soy-based substitute foods
* pasteurized fruit juice
* . . . and so on

2. Eat fruit. This is pretty much the only natural thing you can eat that's sweet—the sweetness that everyone craves (once in a while or constantly) is—on an ancient, instinctive level—about fruit. So eat it, whatever kind you like, as much as you like, as long as it's fresh.

3. Eat fat. It is not healthy to avoid fat at all costs; fat is a vital part of human nutrition. I eat plenty of butter and red meat. If that freaks you out, eat olive oil and avocados, but you need fat. Stop being afraid of it. However, be very afraid of odorless, flavorless vegetable seed fats, hydrogenated fats, and spreads. As a good rule of thumb, your fats should contain one ingredient (no spreads/blends) and they should smell and taste like what they are (peanut oil and olive oil smell like peanuts and olives; soy oil and canola oil smell like nothing).

4. Don't eat industrial additives. You don't need to learn what each one does to you, they're all bad news. You shouldn't be eating food that needs preservatives or additives anyway, fresh food doesn't require that. Don't trust the people who are selling you the food to tell you how good it is for you. 'All natural' and 'no preservatives' are effectively meaningless, and you need to disregard them until you've checked out the ingredient list for

yourself. If it comes wrapped in plastic, you probably want to avoid it.

5. Grains are absolutely not necessary in the human diet. In fact, it isn't possible for people to eat grains without processing them. Animals that eat grains have completely different digestive systems from ours. Our medium-length digestive systems are perfect for fruit and meat. That's what you should eat. I won't tell you that you can't eat grains and be healthy—obviously there are people who do that. But stop thinking of grains as an essential, or even important part of the human diet, because they aren't.

6. Antioxidants are delicate. Get them from the source in real, whole foods, not added into processed foods.

7. Ignore fads/trends. People have the same nutritional needs as they had last week or a hundred years ago. They don't change. Find what works and stick with it.

8. Great protein sources include meat, dairy (full fat), eggs, fish, nuts, seeds, and beans. You'll need it now that you're exercising, so make sure you get it every day.

For a more in-depth look into a simpler and more useful way to understand human nutrition, you may be interested in my book on the subject:

The Natural Diet: Simple Nutritional Advice For Optimal Health In The Modern World by Patrick Barrett

SUPPLEMENTS

It makes sense for this section to come after Basic Nutrition, and if you've read that then you can probably guess what I'm going to say here. I don't take supplements of any kind, and I can't recommend them to you either.

Many people nowadays who spend time lifting weights or participating in sports choose to use any of a number of different supplements. To someone who is just getting started with exercise, it might almost seem like you 'can't' make progress toward your exercise goals without using supplements too.

I can tell you, first of all, that it is absolutely possible to get bigger and stronger without the use of supplements—after all, people have been big and strong since long before these supplements were available. I don't use any supplements, and I have seen great results from my time spent working out.

Having said that, even though supplements in general do not tend to fall in line with the dietary methods I recommend, it is not accurate to say that all supplements are 'evil.'

The best advice that I can give you is to research anything you're thinking of putting into your body. Find out about ingredients, about any potential side effects, look for recommendations from people you trust, and figure out if you think using that product is a good decision.

Whatever choice you make, you need to stick to a healthy, natural diet, and pay close attention to how your body reacts to anything you put into it. Also, always remember the importance of patience. Keep the big picture in mind, and never sacrifice your long-term health for short-term gains.

VITAMINS

Many people take multivitamins, and I won't say that you shouldn't do that, but I will give you a few thoughts about them:

1. The best source of a vitamin or any nutrient is always from real food. Fresh fruit, dairy, nuts, seeds, beans, and meat are loaded with vitamins and minerals, and your body is best at absorbing them from these real foods. No multivitamin can beat a diet that is naturally rich in vitamins.

2. It's hard and unnatural for your body to use vitamins delivered all at once in a dense little capsule. A lot of that is wasted and goes right through you. This can be a problem particularly if you adapt the attitude that you don't need to worry about your vitamin intake because you take a multivitamin; then, you think you're covered by the pill (you're probably not) and you don't make up for it with real food, which is not a good situation.

3. If you do take a multivitamin, take one with a reasonable amount of each nutrient (not 10,000% of everything). Always eat it with a meal, and if there are multiple pills space them out during the day, with food, to give your digestive tract a more natural experience (unless, of course and as always, a doctor advises otherwise). If you're going to stray from the natural path of getting your vitamins from your diet, at least simulate a natural experience by not overdoing the doses, by eating them with an actual meal, and by spacing out multiple pills.

4. Also, if you take a vitamin supplement, eat like you don't. In other words, still make sure that you eat an abundance of vitamin-rich foods and don't assume that your multi-vitamin will cover you—think of the multivitamin as an emergency backup, not a primary strategy.

5. Again, disregard everything I just said if a doctor tells you otherwise. Always follow your doctor's advice over mine.

One other important note—women who think they may be pregnant or may become pregnant, intentionally or otherwise, should take folic acid a.k.a. folate a.k.a. vitamin B9 daily. This is present in a lot of healthy foods, so you should be getting it anyway, but if a mother doesn't consume enough early in the pregnancy (and actually right before pregnancy as well), the baby can suffer significant and terrible defects. Some foods that contain folic acid include spinach and other leafy greens, beans, peas, lentils, egg yolks, many fortified grain products, orange juice, grapefruit juice, bananas, and other fruits and vegetables. Better safe than sorry.

WORKING OUT WITH A PARTNER

This is one easy step you can take to drastically increase your workout results. People who have workout partners tend to exercise much more often and more consistently, and see better results. If you have a spouse, sibling, parent, or friend who is also interested in getting into better shape I would seriously consider finding out if he or she is interested in working out with you on a regular basis.

Don't expect to be able to force anybody to exercise with you though—if you find that you have to plead with the person to exercise with you, it kind of kills the whole point of having a partner. The purpose of partnering is that you are able to keep each other motivated and on track, to spot each other, to push each other to do better, and, sometimes, honestly, to make it harder to quit. It can be much easier to not show up to exercise if nobody expects you, as opposed to having to call someone and cancel.

Try to find someone who will be enthusiastic and supportive, someone who you will enjoy exercising with.

You will probably find yourself making much better progress than you would on your own.

There is a potential negative aspect to this though—if your workouts become social sessions where the focus is on talking or hanging out instead of exercise, then that will obviously be a problem. Be careful in choosing your partner, and make sure that your partner—and you—focus on the task at hand and save socializing for later.

CONCLUSION

You now have everything you need to develop and maintain a course of bodyweight training that will help you get stronger, build muscle, lose weight, and maintain healthy joints. The single most important thing now is that you pick a schedule and follow it consistently. Your body was made to exercise, and as long as you perform strenuous exercise on a regular basis, you will be happy with your results, and you will enjoy lifelong strength and health.

Follow a workout schedule that incorporates all the major muscle groups of your body, get quality food and rest while you recover, and then repeat. If you can do that on a regular basis—from now on—you'll be as fit, strong, and healthy as anyone.

BOOKS BY PATRICK BARRETT

Natural Exercise: Basic Bodyweight Training and Calisthenics for Strength and Weight-Loss

The Natural Diet: Simple Nutritional Advice For Optimal Health In The Modern World

ABOUT THE AUTHOR

Patrick Barrett has been interested in exercise ever since he started to lift weights with his dad and older brothers as a kid. He participated in a half-dozen organized sports (most notably inline hockey and high school wrestling) until a neck injury during a wrestling match in his junior year prevented him from playing further in any contact sports.

After the injury, he developed an interest in pursuing strength and balance, particularly through bodyweight and self-taught gymnastic-type exercises.

Patrick has always loved both cooking and eating food. Unsatisfied with the confusing and often contradictory nutritional advice offered by mainstream sources, Patrick searched for another way to understand human nutrition that was logical, consistent, and effective. His books on food and nutrition reflect this 'cleaner,' more intuitive and useful understanding of food and how it impacts our health.

Patrick hopes that his books will save his audience time and aggravation by finally offering practical ways to achieve their nutrition and fitness goals.

19457829R00055

Made in the USA
San Bernardino, CA
27 February 2015